Monkeypox

A threat to health
(declared by public health)

By Laura Norda

Chapter 1: Brief history

Two outbreaks of a disease resembling the pox in colonies of monkeys maintained for a study led to the discovery of monkeypox in 1958. Despite being called "monkeypox," the disease's origin is still a mystery. However, the virus may be carried by African rodents and non-human primates (such as monkeys) and infect humans.

In 10 African nations, the infectious pox virus that causes fever, chills, and rashes is endemic, or persistently regionally prevalent. The fact that HPV was formerly uncommon in Europe and the Americas, however, has traditionally caused Western public health experts to ignore the spread of the disease abroad.

In 1970, the first instance of monkeypox in a person was noted. Monkeypox cases have been documented before the 2022 epidemic in several central and western African nations. Before until recently, practically all occurrences of monkeypox in individuals outside of Africa were connected to either imported animals or foreign travel to nations where the illness often occurs. These incidents happened on many continents.

Monkeypox, which is said to have been around for thousands of years, is shrouded in myth. Even the disease's name is somewhat misleading since rodents are assumed to be the primary host of the illness, with monkeys (and humans) serving as accidental hosts. In a recent publication outlining the need for a non-discriminatory, non-stigmatizing term for the illness, more than 20 experts argued that even if monkeypox is more prevalent in central and western Africa, it is deceptive to refer to the virus as "being African." (Monkeypox will soon have a name change to better reflect this goal.) In actuality, uneven access to the world's vaccine stockpiles and healthcare resources is primarily to blame for the virus's continuing existence in Africa.

Oyewale Tomori, a virologist at Redeemer's University and a former president of the Nigerian Academy of Science, reminds people that the first instance of monkeypox was discovered in a laboratory in Denmark, not in Africa.

Chapter 2: Outbreak

The most recent two cases before the current epidemic were in tourists who returned from Nigeria in 2021. (to Maryland and Texas). A US citizen who had taken two commercial flights to and from Nigeria was the subject of the Texas lawsuit. 200 connections were found via contact tracing, however, no one had any symptoms.

A total of 71 cases of human monkeypox were discovered between May 2003 and July 2003 in six Midwestern states, including Wisconsin (39 instances), Indiana (16), Illinois (12), Kansas (1), Missouri (2), and Ohio (1).

Three kinds of African rodents (Gambian pouched rat, dormice, and rope squirrels) that were brought into the country on April 9, 2003, by a Texas-based importer of exotic pets were found to be the source of the epidemic. These were sent from Texas to a distributor in Illinois, who kept them alongside prairie dogs, which later contracted an infection.

The epidemic was the first occurrence of monkeypox infection in the Western Hemisphere and the United States. There were no recorded fatalities and no evidence of human-to-human transmission. Direct contact with infected prairie dogs was a factor in each instance. Electron microscopy, polymerase chain reaction, and immunohistochemical tests were utilized to demonstrate that human monkeypox was the causal culprit.

In nations where the virus is "endemic," such as the Central African Republic, Democratic Republic of the Congo, Liberia, Nigeria, Republic of the Congo, and Sierra Leone, confirmed cases of monkeypox have risen since 2016. In Nigeria, an epidemic of more than 80 cases occurred that year.

The rate of human-to-human transmission has often been low.

For instance, attack rates were relatively high in families during an epidemic of monkeypox in the Democratic Republic of the Congo (reported in 2016); the region's declining immunity to smallpox is very much a risk factor in the DRC.

More than 100 cases of monkeypox have been reported to the World Health Organization since May 13, 2022, as part of an ongoing epidemic in non-endemic areas. Spain, Portugal, the United Kingdom (where the first European case was documented), Belgium, France, Germany, Italy, Sweden, Australia, and Canada have seen the majority of instances worldwide.

Seven confirmed or suspected instances are known to exist in the United States as of this writing: one each in Massachusetts, New York, Florida, Florida, Utah, Washington State, and California.

Many of the instances involve males between the ages of 30-55 who have sex with men, and they may be connected to two sizable raves that were conducted in Belgium and Spain. It should be noted that sexual transmission of monkeypox has never been documented, and transmission is still believed to occur through respiratory droplets during close contact, although lesions have sometimes been discovered in the vaginal and anal areas.

Chapter 3: Causes & Transmission

Monkeypox is caused by the orthopox virus. The lipoprotein layer has tubules or filaments that cover the viral DNA, and the viruses are oval brick-shaped. This viral genus is made up of several species, including variola (smallpox), cowpox, buffalopox, camelpox, rabbitpox, and others. The majority of species only infect one kind of animal, however rarely they may also infect other animals.

Monkeypox is mostly spread by direct contact with sick animals, while it is also possible to get the disease by consuming undercooked meat from infected rodents or monkeys. Particularly when the human skin is torn due to bites, scratches, or other trauma — these are possible causes of viral infection. Cutaneous or mucosal sores on the infected animals are a likely route of transmission to humans. Although it is not often reported, human-to-human transmission, likely via contaminated respiratory droplets, is a possibility. The most probable means of transmission include direct skin contact with lesions, bodily fluids, and contaminated bedding or clothing. According to one research, just 8% to 15% of illnesses were spread from person to person among immediate family members.

There are many ways that monkeypox spreads.

Anyone may get monkeypox via close, direct, and often skin-to-skin contact, including:
Direct touch with a monkey-pox patient's rash, scabs, or bodily fluids.

interacting with items, materials (such as clothes, beds, or towels), or surfaces that have been touched by a person who has monkeypox.

exposure to respiratory secretions

This direct contact may occur during intimate interactions, such as oral, anal, and vaginal intercourse, as well as when someone has monkeypox and you touch their genitalia (penis, testicles, labia, and vagina), massages, kisses, and hugs.

extended face-to-face interaction,

by touching linens, towels, and fetish equipment that have not been cleaned and were previously used by a person who has monkeypox.

Through the placenta, a pregnant individual may transmit the virus to their unborn child.

Additionally, individuals may get monkeypox from diseased animals by being bitten or scratched by them, preparing or consuming meat from them, or using their products.

From the moment symptoms appear until the rash has completely disappeared and a new layer of skin has developed, a person with monkeypox might transmit it to others. Usually, the disease lasts two to four weeks.

Chapter 4: Signs & Symptoms

Monkeypox symptoms might include:
- Fever
- Headache
- Back pain and muscle aches
- Enlarged lymph nodes
- Chills
- Exhaustion
- respiratory issues (e.g., sore throat, nasal congestion, or cough).
- a rash that appears on or near the genitalia (penis, testicles, labia, and vagina) or anus (butthole), but can also appear on the hands, feet, chest, face, or mouth

Before the rash heals, it will go through several phases, including scabs.

The rash may feel uncomfortable or itchy and may resemble pimples or blisters.

You could just encounter a few or all of the symptoms.

Sometimes the rash appears first, then the accompanying symptoms. Some people merely get a rash.

Monkeypox often results in a rash.

Some patients have a rash that appears before (or independently of) other symptoms.

After being exposed to the virus for three weeks, monkeypox symptoms often appear. When experiencing flu-like symptoms, a rash often appears 1–4 days later.

Until the rash has healed, all scabs have come off, and a new layer of skin has developed. Monkeypox may be transmitted from person to person. Usually, the disease lasts two to four weeks.

Not everyone who has monkeypox typically has all of the symptoms. Many patients in the current (2022) epidemic aren't exhibiting the typical constellation of symptoms. Only a few lesions, no enlarged lymph nodes, a lower fever, and fewer additional symptoms of sickness are present in this unusual presentation. You may possess it without realizing it. However, even if you don't exhibit many symptoms of an illness, you may still infect others via extended close contact.

If You Have Any Other Symptoms, Including a New or Unexplained Rash, avoid becoming intimate or having close contact with anybody until you have been examined by a healthcare professional.
Visit a community health center in your area if you don't have a doctor or health insurance.
Wear a mask and let the doctor or nurse know that the virus is active nearby when you visit them.

Chapter 5: Prevention

Follow these instructions to avoid contracting monkeypox:

- Do not come in close contact with somebody who has a rash that resembles monkeypox.
- Never touch a monkeypox victim's rash or sores.
- Avoid sharing intercourse, kissing, hugging, and cuddling with someone who has monkeypox.
- Avoid coming into touch with items and materials that a monkeypox victim has used.
- Sharing cups or eating utensils with someone who has monkeypox is not advised.
- Never handle or touch a person who has monkeypox's bedding, towels, or clothes.
- Use an alcohol-based hand sanitizer or often wash your hands with soap and water, particularly after using the restroom and before touching your face or eating.
- Avoid interacting with rodents and primates in Central and West Africa since they are the main carriers of the monkeypox virus.
- Avoid touching bedding or other items that ill or dead animals have touched, as well as sick or dead animals.

Vaccine

Vaccination is advised for those who have been exposed to monkeypox and for those who may be at higher risk of contracting the disease.

Those who are more susceptible to monkeypox include:
- People who have been recognized as contacts of a monkeypox case by public health agencies,
- People who are aware that one of their sexual partners has had monkeypox over the preceding two weeks
- Those who had many sexual partners over the previous two weeks in a region where monkeypox is known to exist
- People who may be exposed to orthopoxviruses due to their occupations include
- Orthopoxvirus testing specialists in laboratories
- Employees in laboratories who handle orthopoxvirus-infected cultures or animals
- a few specially trained healthcare or public health personnel

How can one reduce the danger involved in having sex?
Be mindful of any new or unexplained rashes on your body or your spouse's body, particularly the genitalia and the anus, and discuss any recent illnesses with your partner. Do not have sex and instead see a doctor if you or your partner have recently been unwell, feel sick right now, or have a new or unexplained rash.

The best method to protect yourself and others if you or your partner has monkeypox is to avoid the sexual activity of any type (oral, anal, vaginal), and to avoid kissing or touching each other's bodies while you are ill, particularly if you have any rash. Things like towels, fetish gear, sex toys, and toothbrushes shouldn't be shared.

If you or your partner has monkeypox or suspects they may have it and you want to engage in sexual activity, take into account the following precautions to lessen the risk of the virus spreading:

To minimize skin-to-skin contact, think about having sex while wearing clothing or covering rash-prone regions. Condoms might be helpful if the rash is limited to the genitalia or the anus, but they probably won't be enough to stop monkeypox on their own.

Do not kiss.

After having sex, don't forget to wash your hands, fetish accessories, and any materials (bedding, towels, clothes).
Your risk of contracting monkeypox may rise if you engage in frequent or anonymous intercourse. Your risk of exposure may be decreased by limiting the number of sex partners you have.

Do not touch the rash. Touching the rash increases the risk of it spreading to other areas of the body and slows recovery.

What should a person do if they have additional symptoms or a new, unexplained rash?
Wait until you've been examined by a healthcare professional before engaging in any sexual activity or personal contact.
Visit a community health center in your area if you don't have a doctor or health insurance.
Wear a mask and let the doctor or nurse know that the virus is active nearby when you visit them.
Avoid social events, particularly if they include intimate, one-on-one interaction.
Consider the individuals with whom you have interacted intimately, personally, or sexually during the last 21 days, including those you met via dating apps. If you have been diagnosed with monkeypox, you could be requested to share this information to assist halt the spread.

How may attendees of raves, parties, clubs, and festivals lessen their risk of contracting monkeypox?
When deciding what to do, look for advice from reliable sources like your community's health department.
Second, think about how much intimate, one-on-one interaction and skin-to-skin contact are likely to happen

at the event you're going to. Do not go to any event if you are feeling ill or have a rash; instead, visit a doctor.

It is safer to attend festivals, gatherings, and concerts if everyone is dressed appropriately and there is less chance of skin-to-skin contact. Attendees should use caution while kissing or engaging in other actions that might transmit monkeypox.

There is some danger while attending a rave, party, or club where there are little clothes and frequent direct, close touch between people's bodies. Consider avoiding any rash you notice on other people and reducing skin-to-skin contact.

Monkeypox may be more likely to spread in enclosed areas like bathrooms, saunas, sex clubs, or both private and public sex parties where numerous people engage in close, often anonymous sexual contact.

Societal settings

A communal living environment may get infected with monkeypox if a staff person, volunteer, or resident with monkeypox resides there.

Congregate living circumstances are defined in this article as residences or other housing where unrelated individuals live nearby and share at least one shared room (e.g., sleeping room, kitchen, bathroom, living room). Congregate living environments may include jails and prisons, homeless shelters, group houses, residence halls at colleges and universities, lodging for seasonal workers, residential drug rehab centers, and other places of the same kind. Although these locations could provide personal care services, they are not standard medical facilities (e.g. hospitals). If medical treatment is offered on-site, it is often done so in designated locations or by outside medical staff (e.g., home health care workers).

If a case of monkeypox has been discovered at a facility for communal living, take the following precautions:
Inform staff, volunteers, and residents on monkeypox prevention, particularly the possibility of transmission via close physical contact, such as sexual activity.
Communicate with employees, volunteers, and residents.
Advise on prevention, including ideas for safer sex.
When discussing monkeypox, stick to fact-based communication to prevent stigma.

Consider taking the following measures to address instances at the facility:
Any employee, volunteer, or tenant who seem to have monkeypox should be examined by a doctor and tested for the disease.
Until all scabs detach and a new layer of healthy skin has developed below, those who have been diagnosed with monkeypox should remain segregated from other people.
The municipal or state health agency should be consulted before deciding whether to stop isolating patients.

Monkeypox-infected employees or volunteers should stay at home until they are completely well.

Policies for sick leave that are accommodating and non-punitive for employees are essential to stopping the spread of monkeypox.

While some congregate living facilities may be able to provide isolation on-site, others would need to relocate individuals for isolation.

A door that may be closed and a separate restroom from the rest of the building should be provided for tenant isolation rooms. Residents with several positive monkeypox tests are permitted to share a room.

Only employees who are necessary for isolation area operations should access the area.

Residents with monkeypox should cover any skin lesions with long trousers and long sleeves, a sheet, or a gown if they need to leave the isolation area and should wear a well-fitting disposable mask over their nose and mouth.

Waste from isolation zones should be handled in compliance with U.S. Department of Transportation (DOT) Hazardous Materials Regulations, including handling, storing, treating, and discarding dirty personal protective equipment (PPE), patient dressings, etc (HMR; 49 CFR, Parts 171-180.)

Depending on the type of monkeypox virus the patient possesses, different waste management procedures and category designations may be necessary.

The West African lineage has been recognized as the case in the present epidemic, and the garbage from these individuals is categorized as controlled medical waste (Category B). For the management, storage, treatment, and disposal of waste, facilities must also adhere to municipal and state laws.

Determine who may have been exposed to the monkeypox.

To identify and keep an eye on the health of any employee, volunteer, or resident who may have been in close contact with someone who has monkeypox, facilities should engage with their state or local health authority. Contact tracing may be used to find those who have been exposed and stop further occurrences. This may not always be possible, however, use exposure risk assessment recommendations to identify those who have a high level of exposure to someone with monkeypox if contact tracing is possible. For those who have had significant levels of exposure, the state or local health agency may provide post-exposure immunization.

Depending on the nature of the location, workers, volunteers, and residents who spent time in the same area as someone with monkeypox in a facility where contact tracing is not possible should be regarded as having intermediate or low degree exposure (e.g. level of crowding). Low or moderate degree exposures do not need post-exposure immunization unless the state or local health authorities deem it essential.

Ensure that there is access to handwashing facilities.

All employees, volunteers, and residents should have free access to soap and water or hand sanitizer that has at least 60% alcohol at all times. Everyone should promptly wash their hands after touching lesions, clothes, linens, or any other items that may have come into contact with lesions.

Clean and sanitize the locations where monkeypox patients frequent. Refrain from using fans, dry dusting, sweeping, or vacuuming in these areas since these actions might spread dried material from lesions.

Use an EPA-registered disinfectant with an Emerging Viral Pathogens claim to perform disinfection; they may be found on the EPA's List Q. Observe the manufacturer's recommendations for handling, contract duration, and concentration. Regular detergent and warm water may be used to wash linens. Soiled clothes should always be confined in a laundry bag and handled carefully to prevent the spread of infectious materials. Mattresses in isolation spaces may be made simpler to clean by being covered (for example, with sheets, blankets, or a plastic cover).

For employees, volunteers, and residents, it is necessary to provide the proper personal protective equipment (PPE). Employers are also responsible for making sure that no person is exposed to dangerous amounts of cleaning and disinfection chemicals. In these situations, personnel, volunteers, or residents should wear PPE:

When entering isolation areas, employees should wear protective gear like a gown, gloves, eye protection, and a particulate respirator that has been approved by NIOSH and has N95-rated filters or higher.

Laundry: Employees, volunteers, or residents should wear a gown, gloves, eye protection, and a properly fitted mask or respirator while handling soiled laundry from patients who have a known or suspected monkeypox illness. PPE is not required after the wash cycle.

Cleaning and disinfection: When cleaning locations where persons with monkeypox have been, employees, volunteers, or residents should use a gown, gloves, eye protection, and a properly fitted mask or respirator.

Uses for Household Disinfection

Those who don't need to be hospitalized but still have monkeypox may be kept home alone. People may get monkeypox directly through an infectious rash, via bodily fluids, or by prolonged face-to-face contact with someone who has it. From the moment the initial symptoms appear until the scabs have parted and the skin has completely recovered, the monkeypox virus may still be transmitted.

Body fluids, respiratory secretions, and lesion material from monkeypox patients may pollute the surroundings while the disease is contagious. Poxviruses may persist in bed linens, clothes, and on environmental surfaces, especially in situations with low humidity, darkness, and temperature. In one case, 15 days after a patient's residence was abandoned, researchers discovered an active virus. According to studies, several closely related orthopoxviruses may survive for weeks or months in an environment resembling a home. In comparison to non-porous (plastic, glass, metal) surfaces, porous materials (bedding, clothes, etc.) have the potential to house live viruses for a longer amount of time.

UV radiation is very sensitive to orthopoxviruses. Despite the ability of orthopoxviruses to persist in the environment, they are also sensitive to a variety of disinfectants, so it is advised to disinfect any spaces (such as a person's home or car) where a person with monkeypox has spent time as well as any objects thought to be potentially contaminated.

Disinfectant: Follow the manufacturer's instructions when using a disinfectant that has received EPA registration. Observe all usage instructions provided by the manufacturer, including those regarding concentration, contact time, and handling. Avoid mixing disinfectants or adding other chemicals, and keep in mind any possible health risks when selecting a disinfectant. To use disinfectants safely and effectively, adhere to the following steps:

Verify your product's EPA registration: On the product, look for the EPA registration number.

Review the instructions: adhere to the product's instructions. To ensure that this is the appropriate product for your surface, check the "use locations" and "surface kinds" sections. Read the "precautionary remarks" after that.

Clean the area beforehand: If the instructions call for pre-cleaning or if the surface is unclean, wash it with soap and water immediately. The disinfectant's effectiveness may be hindered by dirt.

Observe the directions: To ensure the product is effective, the surface should be moist for the specified period. Apply again if required.

People with monkeypox should routinely clean and disinfect the areas they use while in isolation at home to reduce domestic infection.

Isolating alone at home

To prevent household infection, individuals with monkeypox who are isolated alone at home should routinely clean and disinfect the areas they inhabit, especially frequently touched surfaces and things. Afterward, wash your hands with soap and water or an alcohol-based hand rub (ABHR) containing at least 60% alcohol, if one is not readily accessible.

People with monkeypox who are isolated in a household with people who don't have monkeypox should abide by the isolation and infection control recommendations, and any shared areas, furnishings, or other things should be cleaned and disinfected right after use.

Those who have recovered from monkeypox and whose time of seclusion is finished should thoroughly sanitize every area of the house where they had been in touch. To reduce the risk of infection to other family members once you recover, follow these procedures.

If someone other than the person with monkeypox cleans and disinfects, that person should wear, at the very least, disposable medical gloves and a respirator or well-fitting mask.

Wear normal clothes that completely cover the skin, and then wash them right away using the guidelines listed below.

If an ABHR is not accessible, wash your hands with soap and water afterward.

Concentrate your efforts on cleaning any objects or surfaces that came into touch with the monkeypox patient's skin directly or often while they were there. Cleanse if in doubt.

Avoid sweeping or dry dusting to prevent the transmission of infectious particles.

The use of moist cleaning techniques, such as mopping and disinfectant wipes and sprays, is recommended.

Using a vacuum with a high-efficiency air filter is allowed for vacuuming. If a mask or respirator isn't available, make sure the person vacuuming wears one.

In this order, disinfect and clean the home:

encompassing waste in general

Any contaminated waste, such as bandages, paper towels, food packaging, and other everyday garbage, should be gathered and contained in a zippered container.

Laundry: Before cleaning anything else in the room, gather any contaminated clothes and linens. Shaking the linens might transmit infectious particles, so refrain from doing so.
household goods and hard surfaces
Other soft furnishings and upholstered furniture
Flooring and carpet
Waste management

Towels, other fabric goods, used or contaminated clothes, and linens and beds should all be stored until laundry. Monkeypox patients should handle and wash their dirty clothes whenever feasible. The laundry shouldn't be combined with that of other household members.

Use the following washing techniques:

- Utilize best procedures while handling dirty laundry to prevent contact with any contaminants from any rashes that may be visible on the clothing.
- Never shake or handle soiled clothing in a way that might spread infectious particles.
- Laundry rooms in homes

- ☐ Transfer dirty clothing to be washed in a sealable bag or container that may be cleaned afterward. An alternative is to use a cloth bag that can be washed with contaminated objects.
- ☐ Use detergent and wash your clothes as directed on the label in a typical washing machine. Although they are not required, laundry sanitizers may be utilized.
- ☐ Lack of available washing facilities at home:
- ☐ In the absence of in-home washing facilities (those not shared with other homes), people should consult their regional public health office to decide on the best choices for laundering.
- ☐ rocky surfaces (and non-porous car interiors)
- Follow the manufacturer's instructions when routinely cleaning and disinfecting frequently touched objects and surfaces (like light switches or counters).
  - ☐ Tables, worktops, door knobs, toilet flush handles, faucets, light switches, and flooring are examples of surfaces that fall within this category.
  - ☐ Include any inside cabinet areas, drawers, or surfaces of the refrigerator, freezer, or other appliances, if the monkeypox victim has reached them.

- [ ] It is not necessary to disinfect objects or surfaces in the house that are likely to have avoided touch with the individual who is ill with monkeypox.
- [ ] This includes clothes and objects in closets and boxes that haven't come into direct touch with or been around a person who has monkeypox.
- [ ] Wash filthy dishes and dining utensils by hand with hot water and dish soap or in the dishwasher with detergent and detergent.
- [ ] Carpet, soft furnishings, and upholstered furniture (and porous car interiors)
- [ ] Steam cleaning may be an option if the individual who had monkeypox had direct skin contact or significant fluid drainage from rashes onto soft items, including upholstered furniture, carpets, rugs, and mattresses.
- [ ] For further information, consult with state or local health authorities.
- [ ] If the individual who had monkeypox had little to no touch with soft furniture, clean the area with a disinfectant made for that kind of surface.

Waste Management

In general, regular waste management procedures should apply to all residences, even those of monkeypox sufferers who are at home alone. Municipal waste management systems can safely collect and discard waste from people who have infectious diseases by following the established procedures.

The room where they are isolated should have a special, lined garbage can for the individual with monkeypox to use.

Gloves, bandages, and other waste materials and disposables that have come into touch with skin should be packed in a plastic bag before being discarded in the designated trash container.

When removing garbage bags, handling, and disposing of trash, the individual with monkeypox or other family members should use gloves.

If cleaning services are hired, trash should be handled and/or disposed of in compliance with any relevant state, municipal, tribal, and territorial waste management rules and regulations. In Appendix F-2 of the federal interagency advice for handling solid waste contaminated with a Category A infectious material, the Department of Transportation contains information relevant to monkeypox.

Animals and Monkeypox

Individuals with the monkeypox virus can infect animals through intimate contact, such as caressing, snuggling, embracing, kissing, licking, sharing sleeping quarters, and sharing meals with infected animals. Infected animals may also convey the illness to people.

To stop the virus from spreading, people with monkeypox should stay away from pets, domestic animals, and wild animals. If your animal companion has had monkeypox:

Do not give up, put to death, or leave animals only because you fear exposure to the monkeypox virus
Avoid using hand sanitizer, counter cleaning wipes, alcohol, hydrogen peroxide, or other products, such as industrial or surface cleaners, to wipe or bathe your pet.
Ask friends or family who reside in a different home to look after the animal while the person with monkeypox is recovering if they did not have close contact with pets after the onset of symptoms. Petting, caressing, embracing, kissing, licking, sharing sleeping spaces, and sharing meals are all examples of close contact.

Clean your house once the individual who had monkeypox healed before introducing healthy animals inside.

For 21 days following the most recent contact, pets that were near a person who had monkeypox symptoms should be kept at home and away from other animals and people. Care of exposed dogs should not be performed by infected persons. When feasible, ask a family member to take care of the exposed animal until the person with monkeypox recovers. The person with monkeypox should avoid close contact with the exposed animal.

In rare situations, it may be important to isolate and care for animals that have been exposed to monkeypox in a place other than the house. For example, people who are immunocompromised, pregnant, have young children present (<8 years of age), or with a history of atopic dermatitis or eczema, should not provide care for animals that had close contact with a person with monkeypox as they may be at increased risk for severe outcomes from monkeypox disease.

If you have monkeypox and must care for your healthy pets while in home isolation, wash your hands before and after or rub them with an alcohol-based hand rub. While caring for your animals, it's also crucial to wear gloves, a well-fitting mask or respirator, and to cover any skin rashes as much as you can (long sleeves, long pants).

Your pet should not wear a mask.
Keep your distance from your pet.
Ensure your pet cannot mistakenly come in contact with infected objects in the house such as clothes, bedding, and towels used by the person with monkeypox.
Do not allow animals to come in contact with rashes, bandages, and bodily fluids.
Make sure that any food, toys, bedding, or other supplies you provide your animal while it is being isolated don't come into touch with exposed skin or a rash.

What to do if a pet exhibits monkeypox symptoms

While we do not know all the symptoms infected animals may have, observe the animal for possible indicators of disease including lethargy, loss of appetite, coughing, nasal secretions or crust, bloating, fever, and/or pimple- or blister-like skin rash. Call your veterinarian if you discover an animal that seems unwell within 21 days of having contact with a human who has probable or proven monkeypox. Your state's public health veterinarian or animal health official can be informed with the assistance of a veterinarian.

If you suspect your pet has monkeypox, follow these steps:

If your pet has recently developed a rash or two other clinical signs and has been in close contact with someone who has monkeypox, whether it is probable or confirmed, get them tested. If an animal seems sick within 21 days of coming into contact with someone who has monkeypox, whether it be probable or confirmed, call your veterinarian.

As previously mentioned, lethargy, lack of appetite, coughing, bloating, nasal and/or eye secretions or crust, fever, and/or pox-like skin lesions (which may initially resemble a pimple or blister before progressing to a characteristic monkeypox lesion) or rash are all possible clinical signs of monkeypox in animals.

Reduce direct contact with humans for at least 21 days after being ill or until completely healed, and keep the sick pet or animal apart from other animals.

It is best to keep sick animals within their own homes, away from people who haven't had monkeypox, and in isolation.

When caring for sick animals that have had intimate contact with a human who has monkeypox, those who are immunocompromised, pregnant, have small children present (under 8 years of age), or who have a history of atopic dermatitis or eczema, should not do so.
Use personal protection equipment (PPE) and often wash your hands while tending to and cleaning up after ill animals. PPE comprises wearing gloves, employing eye protection (safety glasses, goggles, or face shield), wearing a well-fitting mask or respirator (preferably a disposable NIOSH-approved N95 filtering facepiece respirator), and wearing a disposable gown.
If a disposable gown is not available, wear clothing that completely covers the skin (i.e. long sleeves, long trousers), and promptly remove and clean clothes following contact with the animal, animal enclosures, or animal bedding.
Carefully remove PPE to prevent self-contamination.
After removing PPE, massage your hands together with an alcohol-based product or wash your hands with soap and water.
Guidelines for disposing of garbage may be obtained from your local public health agency, but typical safety measures include:
Use a designated, lined garbage container for any possibly hazardous rubbish.

Do not leave or dispose of rubbish outside since Monkeypox virus infections in animals may develop.
If accepted for the species and your plumbing infrastructure, flush animal excrement down the toilet.
To avoid contaminating humans or other animals, including wild animals and home pests like mice and rats, disposable animal housing, disposable rodent bedding, and animal feces that cannot be flushed down the toilet should be wrapped in a bag and disposed of appropriately.

Bedding, enclosures, food dishes, and any other items in direct contact with infected animals must be properly disinfected following the Disinfecting Home and Other Non-Healthcare Settings.
Bedding and dirty clothes shouldn't be handled in a way that could spread infectious particles, including disposable rodent bedding.

Chapter 6: Treatment

Typically, monkeypox is a self-limiting illness with symptoms that last between two and four weeks. Monkeypox often resolves on its own without medical intervention. After a diagnosis, your doctor will keep an eye on your health, attempt to alleviate your symptoms, avoid dehydration, and provide antibiotics to treat any developing secondary bacterial infections.

For infections caused by the monkeypox virus, there are no particular therapies. However, since the monkeypox and smallpox viruses share genetic characteristics, antiviral medications and vaccinations created to guard against smallpox may also be used to treat and prevent infections with the monkeypox virus.

People who are more prone to get very sick, such as individuals with compromised immune systems, may be advised to take antivirals such as tecovirimat (TPOXX).

Even if you don't believe you have had contact with someone who has the disease, you should see your doctor if you get symptoms of monkeypox.